Copyright ©

Table of contents

Introduction

It's no secret that the human body is impressive. But did you know that trillions of living microorganisms are working behind the scenes to keep you healthy?

Sometimes, those microorganisms need help. Probiotics have been the go-to when it comes to maintaining your body's microbiome, but postbiotics are gaining traction as the new influencer of your microbiome.

What You Should Know About Your Microbiome

Your body's microbiome is a delicate system of "good" and "bad" microorganisms. They work together to maintain your health. If the balance between good and bad microorganisms is imbalanced, you'll feel it.

The organisms in your microbiome are bacteria, fungi, viruses, and protozoa. Every person has a different combination of microorganisms, so your microbiome is unique. This uniqueness makes treating problems with your microbiome difficult.

Dysbiosis. An imbalance in your microbiome, or dysbiosis, can have severe complications. Dysbiosis can lead to:

- New allergies

- Autoimmune diseases (inflammatory bowel disease or type 1 diabetes)

- Cancer

- Psychiatric disorders

Probiotics. Probiotics are good bacteria. When you get sick, you may have too much bad bacteria. Probiotics help fight the bad bacteria until you feel better.

When you have an imbalance in your microbiome, you can take probiotic supplements to restore balance. A well-balanced diet generally provides enough good bacteria to maintain your microbiome. Make sure your diet is adequate before seeking supplements.

Prebiotics. The microorganisms in your body need to eat. Probiotics feed on prebiotics, complex carbohydrates such as inulin, pectin, and starches.

Postbiotics. Postbiotics are a byproduct of probiotics when they eat prebiotics. Their goal is the same: maintain your microbiome.

Postbiotics achieve their goal with more control and fewer risks compared to probiotic supplements.

Factors that affect your microbiome. For most people, their microbiome is a stable balance. Your unique microbiome, age, diet, and environmental factors can influence your microbiome's stability. You can use probiotics and postbiotics to restore your microbiome's balance.

What Are Postbiotics?

Don't forget that microorganisms in your microbiome are living. Postbiotics are substances produced by your microorganisms while they go about their business. These substances are not live microorganisms, but they are still beneficial to your microbiome.

Postbiotics are bioactive compounds produced by food-grade microorganisms during a fermentation process—specifically, when the "good bacteria" in your gut digests and breaks down portions of dietary fiber and prebiotics, which are typically found in complex plant carbohydrates. A natural byproduct of this process is the production of short chain fatty acids . And just like probiotics, postbiotics work behind-the-scenes to support gut health

Other names for postbiotics. You may see postbiotics referred to by different names. Some of these names include:

- Paraprobiotics
- Non-viable microbial cells
- Fermented infant formulas (FIFs)

What Are the Benefits and Risks of Postbiotics?

Health benefits. The health benefits of postbiotics aren't fully understood, but they tend to mimic the health benefits of probiotics. Postbiotics:

- Support your immune system.
- Prevent inflammation.
- Have anticarcinogenic qualities.
- Are antimicrobial and prevent infections.
- Can lower the risk of cardiovascular events.
- Can support oxytocin formation, which helps heal wounds and supports birthing functions.

One of the benefits of postbiotics compared to probiotics is the risks involved. Since postbiotics don't contain microorganisms, there's a lower risk of complications from adding new bacteria to your microbiome.

Probiotics are safe for most people. But people with weak immune systems, severe illness, or recovering from surgery can get an infection from probiotics.

Practical benefits of postbiotics. The production of postbiotics is more economical than probiotics. Postbiotics:

- Have a long shelf-life
- Are easily stored
- Are easily transported
- Aren't as sensitive to cold temperatures
- Can be more reliably produced

Are You Considering Postbiotics?

You can get postbiotics from food or supplements. Supplements can be harmful to some people. Before buying probiotic or postbiotic supplements yourself, talk with your doctor.

Genetics, environment, age, medication, and more determine the bacteria in your microbiome. Supplements and certain diets may not be suitable for you, but certain foods can increase the postbiotics in your microbiome.

Gradually change your diet. The best way to balance your microbiome is through a well-rounded diet. If you feed the right foods to your probiotic bacteria, they'll produce postbiotics for you.

If you're able, eating a high-fiber diet can improve your microbiome. Whole fruits, vegetables, legumes, and grains are significant sources of fiber.

Additionally, the following foods contain prebiotics, which feed your microbiome:

- Garlic

- Onions

- Leeks

- Asparagus

- Bananas

- Seaweed

When changing your diet, introduce new foods slowly. Eating too many prebiotic foods can cause gas and bloating. People with gastrointestinal conditions should be cautious with drastic diet changes.

Eating foods with probiotics won't necessarily increase the postbiotics in your body, so be careful when adding probiotic supplements to your diet.

Check With Your Doctor

It bears repeating that postbiotics need more research. Studies have shown positive results, but there's still much to learn. Before taking your microbiome into your own hands through postbiotic supplements, talk with your doctor.

Research involving postbiotics, using postbiotics in various formulations to treat several health conditions, is promising but limited. More studies are needed to fully understand the possible benefits and uses of postbiotics.

May Support the Immune System

In a study published in 2022, researchers noted that compounds might promote communication between the gut microbiome and the immune system. The gut microbiome is the balance of "good" and "bad" microorganisms in the gastrointestinal (GI) tract.

Another study published in 2014 found that postbiotics reduced acute infectious episodes and the use of antibiotics in people with recurrent respiratory tract infections.

Helps Reduce Gastrointestinal Distress

Some evidence suggests that postbiotics help alleviate irritable bowel syndrome (IBS) symptoms and chronic unexplained diarrhea. IBS often causes uncomfortable symptoms like stomach cramps, bloating, constipation, and diarrhea.

Helps Manage Atopic Dermatitis Flares
Some evidence suggests that topical postbiotics may alleviate atopic dermatitis symptoms.Atopic dermatitis is

a type of eczema, a skin condition that causes swollen, itchy, and red patches of skin.

People with atopic dermatitis have a weak skin barrier that makes them sensitive to specific allergens and irritants. Atopic dermatitis may sometimes lead to bacterial, fungal, or viral skin infections and scarring.

One review published in 2020 found that a moisturizer made up of postbiotics helped restore the skin barrier and supported the growth of "good" bacteria that protect the skin.9 In another study published in 2022, researchers administered a moisturizer of prebiotics and postbiotics to 396 people with atopic dermatitis. The researchers noted that the moisturizer was effective after three months and had few side effects.

Might Control the Growth of Cancer Cells

Research has found that postbiotics may have anticancer properties. Your body is constantly repairing and creating cells.12 Sometimes, cells grow out of control and form a tumor. Some tumors are benign and not harmful. In contrast, other tumors can be malignant and cancerous. Cancer cells can spread to other body parts, called metastasizing.

According to a study published in 2021, postbiotics help stop the growth of cancer cells. The researchers noted that, in GI cancers, postbiotics might get rid of cancer cells by supporting a process called apoptosis. Apoptosis is the death of unnecessary or malignant cells.12

Helps Control Blood Sugar

Some evidence suggests that butyrate, a short-chain fatty acid, can help control blood sugar levels.High blood sugar is common among people with diabetes. Blood sugar rises if the body makes little insulin or does not respond to insulin as it should. Insulin is a hormone that unlocks cells, allowing sugar from the food you eat to enter your cells.

Typically, your cells store sugar to later use as energy. Without insulin, sugar builds up in the blood. If uncontrolled, high blood sugar can lead to complications, like a weak immune system and frequent infections.

In a study published in 2021, researchers also noted that postbiotics have anti-inflammation properties. Inflammation affects diabetes, so reducing inflammation might help treat the condition.

Has Been Shown To Help Manage Weight

Research has suggested that short-chain fatty acids, which comprise postbiotics, play a key role in weight loss and management.

Overweight and obesity are common risk factors for heart disease, type 2 diabetes, and cancer. Factors like diet, sleep quality, and exercise often affect weight risk. Certain health conditions, medications, and genetics can cause overweight and obesity, too.16

In one review published in 2015, researchers found that short-chain fatty acids can affect appetite and metabolism. According to the researchers, eating sources of prebiotics, like fermentable foods, can help lose weight. Still, most studies have only looked at animals. Research on the effects of short-chain fatty acids on humans is limited.

Might Be Stored Easier Than Probiotics
Postbiotics are more stable than probiotics since they are not live organisms. In other words, postbiotics have

a lengthier shelf life than probiotics. Manufacturers can store postbiotics at higher temperatures than probiotics and store and transport them easily.

Risks of Postbiotics

You may be tempted to skip the go-between and jump directly to a postbiotic supplement. Still, postbiotic supplements are newer than probiotics themselves. There are products on the market that claim to support digestive health and immune function. Still, some experts warn that more research is needed to fully understand the efficacy and safety of postbiotics.

Some experts advise certain people against taking probiotics, such as:

People with weak immune systems

Those who have severe illnesses

People who recently had surgery

In an immune-compromised state, probiotics could cause an infection. Those people may need to avoid postbiotics, as well. Research is limited on whether postbiotics have interactions with certain health conditions.

Consult a healthcare provider if you have a health condition and consider a postbiotic supplement. They may be familiar with the type and form of postbiotic that may fit your needs, how long to use them, and if there are any potential interactions.

Good Sources of Postbiotics

One of the best ways to produce postbiotics in the body is to eat more prebiotic foods that feed probiotics. Prebiotic foods include:

• Apples

• Asparagus

• Bananas

• Cocoa

• Garlic

• Nuts

• Oats

• Onions

• Pulses (e.g., beans, lentils, peas, chickpeas)

Probiotics exist naturally in your body. You can consume some types of probiotics in the form of supplements and certain foods, such as non-pasteurized fermented foods. Fermented vegetables, kefir, kombucha, and miso are also sources of probiotics.

According to the ISAPP, probiotics include live microorganisms that have demonstrated health benefits. As such, not all fermented foods are sources of probiotics. An unpasteurized fermented food may contain live microbes but not meet the probiotic criteria.

WHICH FOODS WILL HELP TO IMPROVE MY GUT HEALTH?

High Fiber Foods: increasing fiber in the diet is an absolute must. Few sources are: chia seeds, nuts, legumes, cruciferous veggies (cabbage, cauliflower, broccoli, Brussels sprouts), berries (raspberries, blueberries, and blackberries), and winter squash (butternut squash and acorn squash).

Prebiotic foods: besides the high fiber foods mentioned above, other pro-biotic rich foods include asparagus, garlic, onion, Jerusalem artichokes, chicory, oats, leeks, bananas (that are less ripe and more green), Dandelion greens, and spinach.

Probiotic foods: Most probiotic foods are fermented foods that contain living organisms. These include kefir, kimchi, tempeh, miso, kombucha, yogurt, sauerkraut, and sourdough bread.

Anti-inflammatory foods: these foods play a natural role in reducing inflammation and providing anti-inflammatory pathways promoting the health of our gut! These foods include salmon, flax seeds, chia seeds, berries, tomatoes, peppers, broccoli, ginger root, spices like turmeric, and walnuts.

Healthy diet recipes for the gut

Spinach, Lima Bean & Crispy Pancetta Pasta

Ingredients

1 (9 ounce) package fresh spinach pasta

1 tablespoon extra-virgin olive oil

4 ounces diced pancetta

1 (16 ounce) package frozen baby lima beans, thawed

1 cup sliced shallots

2 cloves garlic, minced

½ teaspoon dried rosemary

4 cups baby spinach

3 tablespoons lemon juice

¾ cup grated pecorino cheese, divided

Instructions

• Bring a medium saucepan of water to a boil over high heat. Add pasta and cook according to package directions. Reserve 1 cup of water, then drain the pasta.

• Meanwhile, heat oil in a large skillet over medium-high heat. Add pancetta and cook, stirring occasionally, until crispy, 6 to 8 minutes. Remove with a slotted spoon to a plate. Add lima beans and shallots to the pan. Cook, stirring occasionally, until the shallots are tender, about 3 minutes. Stir in garlic and rosemary; cook, stirring, until fragrant, about 1 minute. Add spinach and cook until wilted, about 2 minutes.

• Add the pasta and the reserved water to the pan. Cook, stirring, until the sauce is thickened, about 1 minute. Stir in lemon juice, the pancetta and half the pecorino. Serve the pasta topped with the remaining pecorino.

Creamy White Chili with Cream Cheese

Ingredients

2 (15 ounce) cans no-salt-added great northern beans, rinsed, divided

1 tablespoon canola oil

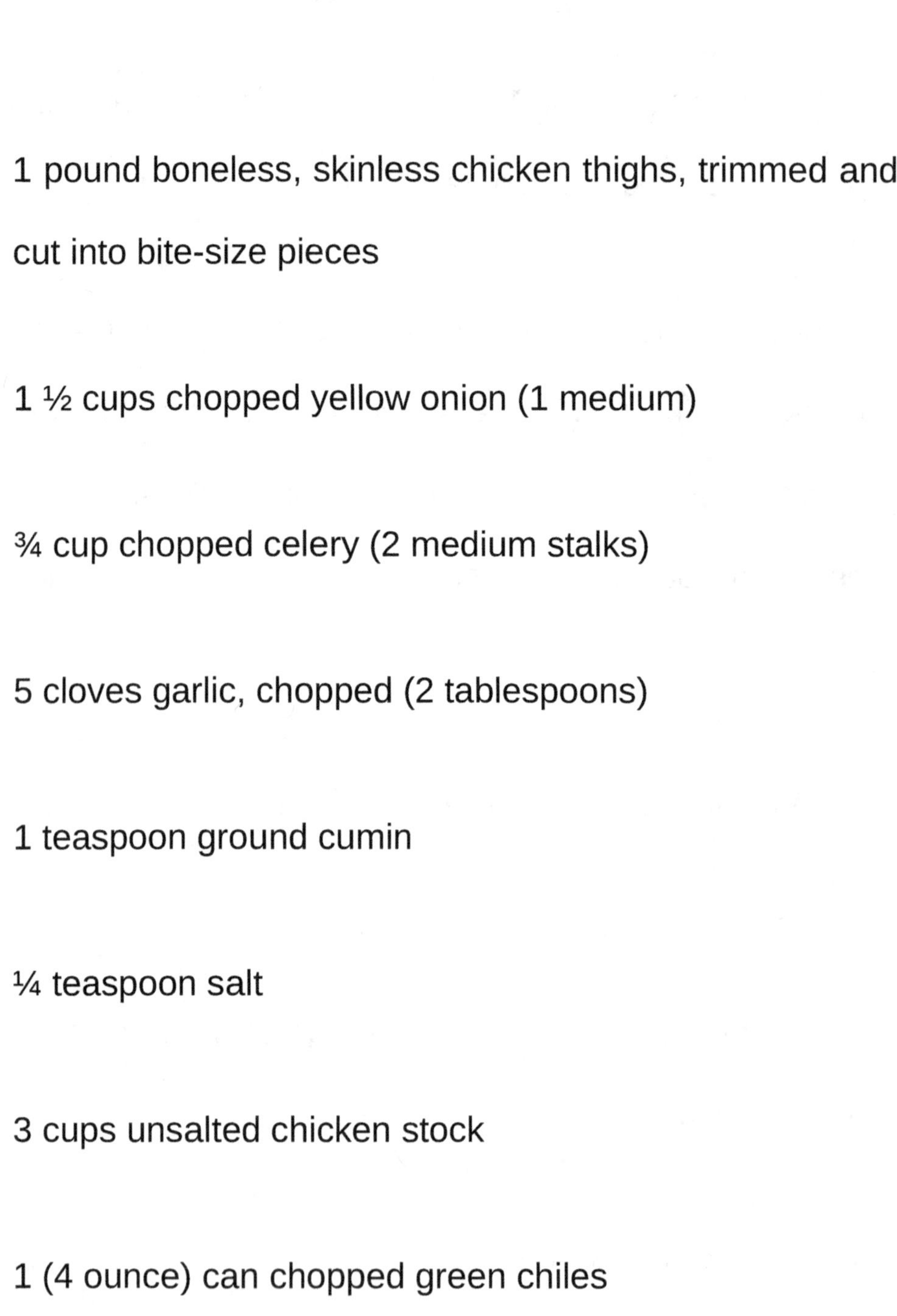

1 pound boneless, skinless chicken thighs, trimmed and cut into bite-size pieces

1 ½ cups chopped yellow onion (1 medium)

¾ cup chopped celery (2 medium stalks)

5 cloves garlic, chopped (2 tablespoons)

1 teaspoon ground cumin

¼ teaspoon salt

3 cups unsalted chicken stock

1 (4 ounce) can chopped green chiles

4 ounces reduced-fat cream cheese

½ cup loosely packed fresh cilantro leaves

Instructions

- Mash 1 cup beans in a small bowl with a whisk or potato masher.

- Heat oil in a large heavy pot over high heat. Add chicken; cook, turning occasionally, until browned, 4 to 5 minutes. Add onion, celery, garlic, cumin and salt. Cook until the onion is translucent and tender, 4 to 5 minutes.

● Add the remaining whole beans, the mashed beans, stock and chiles. Bring to a boil. Reduce heat to medium and simmer until the chicken is cooked through, about 3 minutes. Remove from heat; stir in cream cheese until melted. Serve topped with cilantro

Orange-Mint Freekeh Salad with Lima Beans

Ingredients

2 cups water

¾ cup cracked freekeh (see Tip)

½ cup packed fresh mint leaves, plus more for garnish

½ cup orange juice

3 tablespoons lemon juice

1 small clove garlic, grated

½ teaspoon salt

½ teaspoon ground pepper

¼ cup extra-virgin olive oil

1 cup thinly sliced fennel (1/2 large bulb)

1 cup sugar snap peas, trimmed and thinly sliced

1 cup thinly sliced radishes

2 medium oranges, peeled and segmented

2 cups frozen baby lima beans, thawed

Instructions

- Combine water and freekeh in a medium saucepan and bring to a boil over high heat. Cover, reduce heat to maintain a simmer and cook until the liquid is absorbed, 12 to 15 minutes. Remove from heat and let stand, covered, for 5 minutes. Drain any remaining liquid. Spread the freekeh out on a rimmed baking sheet to cool.

- Meanwhile, combine mint, orange juice, lemon juice, garlic, salt and pepper in a large bowl. Whisk in oil and transfer 1/4 cup of the dressing to a medium bowl. Add fennel, snap peas, radishes and oranges to the medium bowl and toss to combine.

• Add the freekeh and lima beans to the remaining dressing in the large bowl and toss to combine. Serve the fennel mixture over the freekeh mixture. Garnish with more mint, if desired.

White Bean Soup with Pasta

Ingredients

1 tablespoon extra-virgin olive oil

1 ½ cups frozen mirepoix (diced onion, celery and carrot)

2 cloves garlic, minced

1 teaspoon Italian seasoning

1 teaspoon salt

¼ teaspoon crushed red pepper

¼ teaspoon ground pepper

1 28-ounce can no-salt-added diced tomatoes

2 cups low-sodium no-chicken broth or chicken broth

1 15-ounce can low-sodium cannellini beans, rinsed

8 ounces small whole-wheat pasta, such as elbows

1 ½ cups frozen cut-leaf spinach

4 tablespoons grated Parmesan cheese

Instructions

- Put a large saucepan of water on to boil..

- Heat oil in a large pot over medium-high heat. Add mirepoix and cook, stirring, until softened, about 3 minutes. Add garlic, Italian seasoning, salt, crushed red pepper and ground pepper and cook, stirring, until fragrant, about 1 minute. Add tomatoes and their juices, broth and beans and bring to a boil. Reduce heat to maintain a lively simmer. Cover and cook, stirring occasionally, until the tomatoes begin to break down, about 10 minutes.

- Meanwhile, cook pasta in the boiling water for 1 minute less than the package directions. Drain.

- Stir spinach into the soup. Stir in the pasta just before serving. Serve topped with Parmesan.

Black Bean & Slaw Bagel

Ingredients

2 cups shredded green cabbage

2 tablespoons chopped fresh cilantro

2 tablespoons lime juice

⅛ teaspoon salt

½ avocado, mashed

1 jalapeño-Cheddar bagel, halved and toasted

1 cup rinsed no-salt-added canned black beans, heated

Instructions

- Toss cabbage, cilantro, lime juice and salt in a medium bowl. Spread avocado on the top of each bagel half. Top each with 1/2 cup beans and half the slaw.

Black Bean-Cauliflower "Rice" Bowl

Ingredients

1 tablespoon olive oil plus 2 tsp., divided

1 cup frozen cauliflower rice

⅛ teaspoon salt

2 tablespoons chopped onion

2 tablespoons chopped green bell pepper

½ teaspoon chili powder

½ teaspoon ground cumin

¼ teaspoon dried oregano

⅔ cup no-salt-added canned black beans, rinsed

2 tablespoons chopped roasted red pepper

¼ cup water

1 tablespoon lime juice

¼ cup shredded reduced-fat Cheddar cheese

1 medium tomato, chopped

1 tablespoon chopped fresh cilantro for garnish

Instructions

- Heat 1 Tbsp. oil in a medium skillet over medium heat. Add cauliflower rice and salt; cook, stirring often, until heated through, 3 to 5 minutes. Transfer to a small bowl and keep warm. Wipe out the pan.

- Heat the remaining 2 tsp. oil in the pan over medium heat. Add onion, green pepper, chili powder, cumin, and oregano; cook, stirring often, until the vegetables are softened, about 3 minutes. Add beans, roasted red pepper, and water; bring to a simmer. Cook, stirring occasionally, until heated through and thickened, 3 to 5 minutes. Remove from heat. Stir in lime juice.

● Arrange the bean mixture with the hot cauliflower rice in a dinner bowl. Top with cheese and tomato. Garnish with cilantro, if desired.

Vegan Coconut Chickpea Curry

Ingredients

2 teaspoons avocado oil or canola oil

1 cup chopped onion

1 cup diced bell pepper

1 medium zucchini, halved and sliced

1 (15 ounce) can chickpeas, drained and rinsed

1 ½ cups coconut curry simmer sauce (see Tip)

½ cup vegetable broth

4 cups baby spinach

2 cups precooked brown rice, heated according to package instructions

Instructions

• Heat oil in a large skillet over medium-high heat. Add onion, pepper and zucchini; cook, stirring often, until the vegetables begin to brown, 5 to 6 minutes.

• Add chickpeas, simmer sauce and broth and bring to a simmer, stirring. Reduce heat to medium-low and simmer until the vegetables are tender, 4 to 6 minutes. Stir in spinach just before serving. Serve over rice.

Chickpea & Kale Toast

Ingredients

1 tablespoon extra-virgin olive oil

8 cups chopped kale

2 cloves garlic, minced

1 cup rinsed no-salt-added canned chickpeas

Pinch of ground pepper

2 slices whole-grain bread, toasted

½ cup crumbled feta cheese

Instructions

• Heat oil in a large skillet over medium-high heat. Add kale and garlic and cook, stirring occasionally, until soft, about 4 minutes. Stir in chickpeas, salt and pepper. Evenly distribute the mixture between toast slices. Sprinkle with feta

Vegan Black Bean Burgers

Ingredients

1 (15.5 ounce) can no-salt-added black beans, rinsed

1 cup cooked quinoa

½ cup whole-wheat panko breadcrumbs

½ cup chopped scallions

1 tablespoon no-salt-added tomato paste

1 ½ teaspoons ground cumin

½ teaspoon chipotle chile powder

½ teaspoon garlic powder

½ cup vegan mayonnaise, divided

½ teaspoon salt, divided

1 medium avocado

2 tablespoons lime juice

2 tablespoons chopped fresh cilantro

2 tablespoons water

2 tablespoons extra-virgin olive oil

6 small whole-wheat hamburger buns, toasted

6 thin slices tomato

Instructions

- Place beans, quinoa, panko, scallions, tomato paste, cumin, chile powder, garlic powder, 1/4 cup mayonnaise and 1/4 teaspoon salt in a large bowl; mash the mixture together with your hands. Shape into six 3/4-inch-thick patties. Arrange the patties on a plate; refrigerate for 10 minutes.

- Combine avocado, lime juice, cilantro, water and the remaining 1/4 cup mayonnaise and 1/4 teaspoon salt in a food processor; process until smooth, about 30 seconds.

- Heat oil in a large cast-iron skillet over medium-high heat. Add the patties; cook until golden brown, 3 to 4 minutes per side.

- Divide the avocado mixture evenly among top and bottom bun halves. Arrange the bean patties and tomato slices evenly on the bottom bun halves; replace the top bun halves.

Mixed Greens with Lentils & Sliced Apple

Ingredients

1 ½ cups mixed salad greens

½ cup cooked lentils

1 apple, cored and sliced, divided

1 ½ tablespoons crumbled feta cheese

1 tablespoon red-wine vinegar

2 teaspoons extra-virgin olive oil

Instructions

● Top greens with lentils, about half the apple slices and the feta. Drizzle with vinegar and oil. Serve with the remaining apple slices on the side.

Sweet and Savory Hummus Plate

Ingredients

Poached Garlic & Garlic Oil

¾ cup water

4 heads garlic, cloves separate but unpeeled

1 ½ cups canola oil

½ cup extra-virgin olive oil

Bean Dip

1 ½ cups chopped onion

½ teaspoon salt

1 (15-ounce) can cannellini beans, rinsed (see Tip)

1 teaspoon lemon juice

Sweet & Savory Hummus Plate

¾ cup Garlic and White Bean Dip

1 cup green beans or sugar snap peas, stem ends trimmed

8 mini bell peppers

20 Castelvetrano olives

8 small watermelon wedges or 2 cups cubed watermelon

1 cup red grapes

20 gluten-free crackers

1/2 cup salted roasted pepitas

8 coconut-date balls

Instructions

- To prepare poached garlic & garlic oil: Bring water to a boil in a medium saucepan. Remove from the heat, add garlic cloves and stir to submerge. Let stand until the garlic skins are softened and cool enough to handle, about 50 minutes. Strain the garlic, remove the skins and cut off the hard nub where the clove was attached to the head

● Place the garlic, canola oil and olive oil in a medium saucepan; bring to a gentle simmer over medium-low heat. Reduce the heat to low and maintain a very gentle simmer (it may be necessary to slide the pan to the edge of the burner). Simmer until the cloves are golden and very soft when pressed with a fork, 40 to 50 minutes. Let cool for 30 minutes

● Transfer the cooled garlic to a sieve to drain, reserving the oil. Transfer the garlic to a food processor and puree until smooth, scraping down the sides occasionally. (If it makes more than 1/2 cup, store the extra in the refrigerator for up to 1 week.)

• To prepare bean dip: Combine 1/2 cup of the reserved garlic oil, onion and salt in a large skillet. Cook over medium heat until the onion is softened but not browned, 6 to 9 minutes. Stir in beans and cook until heated through, about 2 minutes. Transfer to the food processor, add lemon juice and puree with 1/2 cup garlic puree until smooth. Serve warm or cold. (Store extra garlic oil in the refrigerator for up to 1 week.)

• Divide items equally among 4 plates. If desired, serve with hard cider.

Mixed Greens with Lentils & Sliced Apple

Ingredients

1 ½ cups mixed salad greens

½ cup cooked lentils

1 apple, cored and sliced, divided

1 ½ tablespoons crumbled feta cheese

1 tablespoon red-wine vinegar

2 teaspoons extra-virgin olive oil

Instructions

• Top greens with lentils, about half the apple slices and the feta. Drizzle with vinegar and oil. Serve with the remaining apple slices on the side.

Chipotle Chicken Quinoa Burrito Bowl

Ingredients

1 tablespoon finely chopped chipotle peppers in adobo sauce

1 tablespoon extra-virgin olive oil

½ teaspoon garlic powder

½ teaspoon ground cumin

1 pound boneless, skinless chicken breast

¼ teaspoon salt

2 cups cooked quinoa

2 cups shredded romaine lettuce

1 cup canned pinto beans, rinsed

1 ripe avocado, diced

¼ cup prepared pico de gallo or other salsa

¼ cup shredded Cheddar or Monterey Jack cheese

Lime wedges for serving

Instructions

- Preheat grill to medium-high or preheat broiler.

- Combine chipotles, oil, garlic powder and cumin in a small bowl.

-

- Oil the grill rack (see Tip) or a rimmed baking sheet, if broiling. Season chicken with salt. Grill the chicken for 5 minutes or broil it on the prepared baking sheet for 9 minutes. Turn, brush with the chipotle glaze and continue cooking until an instant-read thermometer inserted in the thickest part registers 165 degrees F, 3 to 5 minutes more on the grill or 9 minutes more under the broiler. Transfer to a clean cutting board. Chop into bite-size pieces.

- Assemble each burrito bowl with 1/2 cup quinoa, 1/2 cup chicken, 1/2 cup lettuce, 1/4 cup beans, 1/4 avocado, 1 tablespoon pico de gallo (or other salsa) and 1 tablespoon cheese. Serve with a lime wedge.

Ginger Veggie Stir-Fry

Ingredients

4 tablespoons vegetable oil, divided

2 teaspoons chopped fresh ginger root, divided

1 ½ cloves garlic, crushed

1 tablespoon cornstarch

1 small head broccoli, cut into florets

¾ cup julienned carrots

½ cup snow peas

½ cup halved green beans

2 ½ tablespoons water

2 tablespoons soy sauce

¼ cup chopped onion

½ tablespoon salt

Instructions

Gather all ingredients.

- Place 2 tablespoons vegetable oil, 1 teaspoon ginger, garlic, and cornstarch in a large bowl; mix until cornstarch is dissolved.

- Add broccoli, carrots, snow peas, and green beans; toss lightly to coat.

- Heat remaining 2 tablespoons vegetable oil in a large skillet or wok over medium heat. Add vegetable mixture and cook for 2 minutes, stirring constantly to prevent burning.

• Stir in water and soy sauce; add onion, salt, and remaining 1 teaspoon ginger. Cook and stir until vegetables are tender but crisp.

• Serve hot and enjoy!

Easy Marinated Artichokes

Ingredients

1 lemon, juiced

2 tablespoons extra-virgin olive oil

2 cloves garlic, chopped (Optional)

1 teaspoon Italian seasoning

1 teaspoon salt, or to taste

1 teaspoon ground black pepper, or to taste

1 (14 ounce) can quartered artichoke hearts, drained

Instructions

● Combine lemon juice, oil, garlic, Italian seasoning, salt, and pepper in a jar. Seal the jar and shake until oil and lemon juice emulsify.

- Remove the lid and add artichoke hearts. Seal again and shake until artichoke hearts are completely coated.

- Serve immediately, or if you like them cold, chill in the refrigerator for at least 1 hour before serving.

Roasted Garlic

Ingredients

10 medium heads garlic

3 tablespoons olive oil

Instructions

- Preheat the oven to 400 degrees F (200 degrees C).

• Arrange heads of garlic on a baking sheet. Sprinkle garlic with olive oil. Bake for 40 minutes to 1 hour, when the garlic is soft and squeezable, it is ready. Remove, let cool, and serve.

Frozen Bananas

Ingredients

4 bananas, peeled and halved horizontally

⅓ cup peanut butter

1 (8 ounce) package semisweet baking chocolate, chopped

½ cup roasted peanuts, chopped

8 ice pop sticks

Instructions

- Insert 1 ice pop stick into the cut end of each banana half. Place the bananas on a wax paper-covered baking sheet, and freeze until the bananas are frozen through, about 2 hours.
- Remove the frozen bananas from the freezer and spread a layer of peanut butter on each banana. Place the peanut butter-covered bananas back in the freezer for 30 to 45 minutes.

- Melt the chocolate in the top of a double boiler over just-barely simmering water, stirring frequently and scraping down the sides with a rubber spatula to avoid scorching.

• Dip each frozen banana in the melted chocolate, spooning the chocolate over the banana to cover it completely. Roll the dipped bananas in the chopped peanuts and place on the wax paper covered baking sheet; freeze until the chocolate is firm, about 1 to 2 hours.

Broccoli, Leek, and Potato Soup

Ingredients

4 slices bacon, diced

2 tablespoons olive oil

3 large leeks, chopped

3 stalks celery, chopped

1 medium onion, chopped

2 tablespoons butter

3 cups chicken stock

3 medium Yukon Gold potatoes, cubed

1 teaspoon herbes de Provence

1 teaspoon ground black pepper

½ teaspoon ground coriander

½ teaspoon fennel seed, crushed

½ teaspoon salt

3 cups broccoli florets

2 ½ cups whole milk

3 green onions, chopped (Optional)

Instructions

● Cook bacon and oil in a large pot over medium heat, stirring occasionally, until bacon is golden brown and has released its grease, about 7 minutes. Add leeks, celery, onion, and butter; cook and stir until leeks have softened, about 7 minutes.

- Add stock, potatoes, herbes de Provence, pepper, coriander, fennel, and salt; increase the heat to high and bring to a boil. Reduce the heat to medium-low, cover, and simmer until potatoes are just beginning to turn tender, about 8 minutes. Stir in broccoli and simmer for 5 minutes. Add milk and continue simmering until vegetables are tender, about 5 more minutes.

- Purée soup with an immersion blender until smooth. Season to taste with salt and pepper. Garnish individual servings with green onions.

Kimchi fried rice

Ingredients

1½ tbsp cold-pressed rapeseed oil

1 garlic clove, sliced

1 thumb-size piece ginger, grated

200g long stem broccoli, chopped

4 spring onions, thinly sliced

50g kimchi

200g pouch wholegrain rice

2 carrots, cut into ribbons using a peeler

2 eggs

1 lime, ½ juiced, ½ as a wedge, to serve

handful coriander

hot sauce, to serve (optional)

Instructions

- Heat 1 tbsp of the oil in a large frying pan, and add the garlic, ginger, broccoli and half the spring onions. Fry for 5-7 mins until softened, then add the kimchi and fry for a couple of mins more. Tip in the rice, breaking it up with the back of your spoon, then stir through the carrot. Cook for a min until all heated through, then push everything to the side of the pan.

- Pour the remaining oil into the empty part of the pan, crack in the eggs, fry to your liking and season. Squeeze the lime juice over the rice and eggs, then scoop the rice into bowls. Top with the egg, coriander leaves, remaining spring onions and hot sauce, if using. Serve with lime wedges.

Healthy salmon bowl

Ingredients

1 tsp rapeseed oil

2 tsp finely chopped ginger

1 large garlic clove, finely chopped

1 pepper (any colour), deseeded and finely chopped

2 fresh or frozen wild salmon fillets (about 80g each; defrosted if frozen)

250g pouch cooked brown rice

4 spring onions, finely sliced

1 small avocado, peeled, halved, stoned and sliced

80g cucumber, halved lengthways and sliced

chilli sauce to serve (optional)

For the miso dressing

4 tbsp kefir

1 tsp white miso paste

1 tsp honey

Instructions

• Heat the oil in a large non-stick pan or deep frying pan with a lid over a medium heat and cook the ginger, garlic and pepper for 2 mins, covered. Stir, then put the salmon on top, cover again and cook for 5 mins until the fish is cooked through.

● Meanwhile, mix the dressing ingredients together in a small bowl. Squeeze the pouch of rice to separate the grains, then tip the contents into a small pan with 2 tbsp water. Cover and cook for 2 mins.

● Stir the spring onions into the rice mixture along with half the dressing. Spoon into two bowls. Remove the skin from the salmon and flake the fish on top of the rice. Top with the pepper, avocado and cucumber, then drizzle over the remaining dressing and some chilli sauce, if using.

Pea & broad bean shakshuka

Ingredients

1 bunch asparagus spears

200g sprouting broccoli

2 tbsp olive oil

2 spring onions, finely sliced

2 tsp cumin seeds

large pinch cayenne pepper, plus extra to serve

4 ripe tomatoes, chopped

1 small pack parsley, finely chopped

50g shelled peas

50g podded broad beans

4 large eggs

50g pea shoots

Greek yogurt and flatbreads, to serve

Instructions

- Trim or snap the woody ends of the asparagus and finely slice the spears, leaving the tips and about 2cm at the top intact. Finely slice the broccoli in the same way, leaving the heads and about 2cm of stalk intact. Heat the oil in a frying pan. Add the spring onions, sliced asparagus and sliced broccoli, and fry gently until the veg softens a little, then add the cumin seeds, cayenne, tomatoes (with their juices), parsley and plenty of seasoning, and stir. Cover with a lid and cook for 5 mins to make a base sauce, then add the asparagus spears, broccoli heads, peas and broad beans, cover again and cook for 2 mins.

• Make 4 dips in the mixture. Break an egg into each dip, arrange half the pea shoots around the eggs, season well, cover with a lid and cook until the egg whites are just set. Serve with the rest of the pea shoots, a spoonful of yogurt and some flatbreads, and sprinkle over another pinch of cayenne, if you like.

Fennel-roasted cauliflower with quinoa

Ingredients

1 large cauliflower, or 2 small ones, separated into florets

1 tbsp fennel seeds

1 tsp coriander seeds

1 tsp smoked paprika

2 tbsp olive oil

1 red onion, chopped

2 peppers (mix of red, yellow or orange), chopped

1 courgette, halved lengthways, cored and chopped

1 small garlic clove, crushed

1 lemon, juiced and zested

4 tbsp yogurt

250g quinoa, cooked

● Heat the oven to 200C/180C fan/gas 6. Bring a large pan of salted water to the boil and cook the cauliflower for 5 mins. Drain and spread out on a surface so any excess water evaporates.

- Crush the fennel and coriander seeds using a pestle and mortar and mix with the paprika and a pinch of seasoning Put the cauliflower in a large bowl, drizzle with half the olive oil and sprinkle over the spice mix. Toss the florets to fully coat them.

- Tip the florets onto a baking tray and space them apart. Put the red onions, peppers and courgettes on a separate baking tray, drizzle with the remaining oil, and cook both for 30-35 mins, turning halfway through so they brown all over and turn slightly crisp in places.

- Mix the garlic with lemon juice and stir through the yogurt, adding a little extra water to loosen if needed.

Stir the roasted onions, peppers and courgettes into the cooked quinoa along with the lemon zest and a pinch of salt.

• Pile the quinoa salad onto a plate, then top with the cauliflower florets. Drizzle over the garlic yogurt.

High-fibre muesli

Ingredients

300g jumbo oats

100g All-Bran

25g wheatgerm

100g dark raisins

140g ready-to-eat apricots, snipped into chunks

50g golden linseed

Instructions

- Mix everything in a large bowl. You can store this for up to 2 months in an airtight container. When you're ready to serve, pour lots of chilled milk over and let it soak for a few minutes.

Apricot & seed protein bar

Ingredients

140g dried apricot

40g oats

40g desiccated coconut

25g sunflower seed

1 tbsp sesame seeds

15g dried cranberries

3 tbsp hemp protein powder

1 tbsp chia seeds

Instructions

- Purée apricots in a food processor with 150ml boiling water and the oats, then scrape the mixture into a bowl. Toast coconut, sunflower seeds and sesame seeds in a non-stick pan over a low heat, then stir into the apricots with the cranberries, hemp powder and chia seeds to make a thick paste.

- Roll into a long log on a sheet of cling film. Wrap tightly, chill, then slice thinly to serve. Will keep in the fridge for 2 weeks.

Banana smoothie

Ingredients

500ml unsweetened almond milk

2 tbsp almond butter

6 prunes

1 tsp cinnamon

1 small ripe banana

Instructions

- In a blender, whizz the almond milk with the almond butter, prunes, cinnamon and banana.

- Transfer to 2 bottles and chill until ready to drink, or pack for lunch on the go. The smoothies will keep in the fridge for 2 days.

Bean & dill pilaf with garlicky yogurt

Ingredients

2 onions, halved and thinly sliced

25g butter

175g basmati rice

20g pack dill, stalks and fronds chopped but kept separate

500ml vegetable stock

300g frozen mixed vegetable, broad beans, peas and green beans

100g Greek yogurt

1 tbsp milk

1⁄2 garlic clove, crushed

Instructions

• Fry the onions in the butter until golden. Add the rice and dill stalks; stir round the pan.

• Pour in the saffron stock, bring to the boil, then cover and simmer for 5 mins. Add the beans and half the dill. Cook 5 mins more until the liquid has been absorbed into the rice. Meanwhile, stir the yogurt, milk and garlic together with seasoning. Spoon yogurt on top of the rice, then sprinkle with remaining dill.

Kefir breakfast smoothie

Ingredients

1 large mango, stoned and chopped

2cm piece ginger, finely grated

½ tsp ground turmeric

200ml fresh orange juice

300ml kefir

1-2 tbsp honey or agave, to taste

Instructions

- Put all the ingredients in a blender and blitz until completely smooth. Taste and add a little more ginger, turmeric and honey, if you like.

- Pour into two tall glasses and serve. Can be chilled in a covered jug in the fridge for up to 24 hrs.

Miso & butternut soup

Ingredients

2 tsp rapeseed oil

1 large onion, chopped

400g butternut squash, skin-on, cut into chunks

2 garlic cloves, chopped

210g can butter beans, drained

2 tsp vegetable bouillon

80g shredded kale, finely chopped

2 tsp sesame oil

2 tsp toasted sesame seeds

2 tsp finely grated ginger

1 tbsp brown rice miso

Instructions

● Heat the oil in a large pan and fry the onion for 5 mins to soften. Add the squash and garlic, and stir for a minute. Add the beans and bouillon along with a litre of water, then cover and simmer for 20 mins until the squash is tender.

- Meanwhile, steam the kale for 10 mins, then toss together with the sesame oil, seeds and ginger.

- Add the miso to the soup, then blitz until smooth using a hand blender. Pour into bowls and top with the sesame kale mix to serve.

Asparagus, avocado & quinoa tabbouleh

Ingredients

300g quinoa

250g soya beans

12 fat asparagus spears, woody ends snapped off and tips and stalks separated

300g Greek yogurt

1 tsp sweet paprika, plus a pinch to serve

2 garlic cloves, crushed

zest and juice 2 lemons

½ large cucumber, halved lengthways, seeds scooped
out with a teaspoon, sliced

4 spring onions (we used the ones with the fat bottoms),
thinly sliced

large pack mint, leaves picked

2 small packs dill, roughly chopped

large pack parsley, roughly chopped

2 avocados, stoned, peeled and cut into chunks

juice 3 limes

1 tbsp agave syrup

2 tbsp rapeseed oil

Instructions

- Cook the quinoa following pack instructions, then leave to cool. Bring a pan of water to the boil, add the soya beans and cook for 2 mins, then add the asparagus tips and cook for 1 min more. Drain everything and leave to cool.

- Meanwhile, mix the yogurt with the paprika, garlic and most of the lemon zest. Season and chill.

- Using a vegetable peeler, slice the asparagus stalks into thin ribbons (you won't be able to do the whole stalk as it will get too thin, but these pieces are perfect for soup.) Keep in iced water until ready so they curl.

• On a large platter, combine the quinoa, cooked soya beans and asparagus tips, cucumber, spring onions, herbs and avocado. Drain the asparagus ribbons and add them too. Whisk together the lime and lemon juices, agave syrup, rapeseed oil and some seasoning, then pour over the salad and gently toss to mix. Serve with the yogurt alongside, topped with the remaining lemon zest.

Cucumber kimchi

Ingredients

500g mini cucumbers, halved lengthways

2 tsp flaky sea salt

1 tsp caster sugar

½ apple, grated

3 cloves garlic, sliced

a thumb-sized piece ginger, shredded

2 tbsp gochugaru, (see notes below)

1 tbsp fish sauce

1 tbsp soy sauce

3 spring onions, shredded

Instructions

• Put the cucumber pieces into a bowl and sprinkle over the salt. Toss and leave for 20 minutes to draw out the moisture, then drain.

● Put the sugar, apple, garlic, ginger, gochugaru, fish sauce and soy sauce into a bowl and mix well. Add in the drained cucumbers and spring onions, and toss really well. Spoon into a shallow dish and leave covered at room temperature for 12 hours or overnight, stirring every now and again. It's then ready to serve or will keep covered in the fridge for a week, with the cucumbers becoming softer and funkier with time.

www.ingramcontent.com/pod-product-compliance
Lightning Source LLC
Chambersburg PA
CBHW061249250726
48653CB00002B/588